Aging with Dignity

Unveiling the Secrets of Timeless Beauty and Grooming

Hardman Torres

Table of Contents

CHAPTER ONE

Introduction

Overview of Aging Grooming and Style

Aging is a part of life and with it comes a variety of changes. As one grows older, the body changes, and so does the way they view themselves and the way they want to present themselves to the world. Aging grooming and style are important aspects of how an individual present themselves and how they want to be perceived by others.

Grooming and style for aging adults is about more than just looking good. It's about feeling good and staying healthy. Grooming can range from basic hygiene habits like showering, brushing teeth and combing hair, to more specific activities like styling hair and manicuring nails. The style of clothes an aging adult wears can be a reflection of who they are and how they want to be seen by others. Aging adults will often opt for more comfortable and loose-fitting clothing that is easier to move in, or clothing that is designed to hide blemishes and wrinkles. Styling oneself in clothing that is flattering and comfortable can help aging adults feel more confident and secure in their own skin. Grooming and styling can also help aging adults stay healthy. Proper hygiene habits and hair care can help prevent infections and disease, while maintaining a healthy diet and exercise routine is important for overall physical health

Finally, grooming and style can help aging adults stay connected with the world around them. By dressing in clothing that is fashionable and modern, aging adults can stay up to date with current trends and remain relevant in the eyes of their peers and family.

Overall, aging grooming and style is an important part of how an individual present themselves and how they want to be perceived by others. It is also an important part of staying healthy and staying connected with the world. By taking good care of themselves and dressing in clothing that is comfortable and flattering, aging adults can feel more confident and secure in their own skin.

Benefits of Grooming and Styling

Grooming and styling are essential aspects of personal care. They provide individuals with a well-groomed appearance, which can have a positive effect on confidence, self-esteem, and overall quality of life. At its simplest, grooming is the practice of caring for one's physical appearance. This includes bathing, brushing one's hair and teeth, trimming nails, and other activities. Styling is the process of modifying one's appearance, typically through clothing, hair, and makeup.

The primary benefit of grooming and styling is improved physical appearance. Regular bathing, brushing, and trimming of nails can help maintain a healthy body. Proper hair and makeup can also enhance one's features and create a polished look. In addition to improving physical appearance, grooming and styling can also improve mental and emotional well-being. Feeling confident and looking good can have a positive effect on self-esteem and overall outlook. For those who struggle with self-image issues, regular grooming and styling can help build confidence and self-worth. Grooming and styling can also signal to other people that you care about yourself and your appearance. This can have positive effects in many areas of life, from job opportunities to romantic relationships.

Finally, grooming and styling are important for hygiene reasons. Regular bathing and proper dental care help to reduce the risk of illness and infection. Trimming nails and maintaining a neat appearance can also help prevent skin irritation, which can be caused by long nails or clothing that is too tight or too loose.

CHAPTER TWO

Grooming Basics

Hair Care

Hair care is a necessary and important part of aging adults' personal care. As people age, their hair may become thinner and more prone to breakage and other issues. Proper hair care is necessary to keep hair healthy and looking its best.

The first step in caring for aging adult hair is to use the right shampoo and conditioner. Aging hair is often drier and more prone to breakage, so it is important to use a shampoo that is specifically designed for aging hair. Look for products that contain ingredients like keratin, panthenol, and proteins, which help to protect and strengthen the hair.

The next step is to use a deep conditioner once or twice a week. Deep conditioners are designed to penetrate the hair shaft, which can help to repair the damage and keep the hair hydrated. Look for products that contain natural moisturizing ingredients like shea butter, coconut oil, and avocado oil. It's also important to use a wide-toothed comb when combing out aging adult hair. Wide-toothed combs are less likely to pull and tug on the hair and cause breakage. Start combing at the ends of the hair and work your way up to the roots.

When it comes to styling, aging adult hair can be more prone to breakage, so it is important to use the right tools and products. Heat styling tools like curling irons and flat irons can cause damage to the hair, so it is best to avoid using them. Instead, opt for products like volumizing mousses and hairsprays that can help to create volume without the use of heat.

Finally, it is important to get regular trims to keep the hair healthy and looking its best. Trimming the ends of the hair regularly can help to prevent split ends and breakage. It is also important to avoid over-styling, as this can cause damage to the hair and lead to breakage.

Hair care for aging adults can be a bit more complicated than for younger adults, but with the right products and a few simple steps, it is possible to keep aging adult hair looking healthy and beautiful.

Skin Care

Skin care is an important part of aging well and maintaining quality of life. As people age, their skin becomes more fragile, prone to dryness and irritation, and more susceptible to injury. Proper skin care can help protect against skin problems and maintain a healthy, vibrant appearance.

The skin of aging adults is thinner, drier and less elastic than younger skin. It is also more vulnerable to environmental damage and injury. The skin's protective barrier functions, such as production of oil and sweat, also decrease with age.

Sun exposure is a major factor in skin aging. Sun damage can lead to wrinkles, age spots and skin cancer. To protect skin from the sun's damaging rays, use a broad-spectrum sunscreen with an SPF of at least 30, and wear protective clothing and hats. Avoid outdoor activities between 10am and 4pm when the sun is strongest.

Moisturizing is an important part of skin care for aging adults. Use a moisturizer with natural ingredients, such as hyaluronic acid, to help retain moisture in the skin. Apply moisturizer immediately after bathing or showering, while the skin is still damp, to help lock in moisture.

Cleansing is also important for aging skin, but it is important to use gentle, non-irritating cleansers. Avoid products with harsh chemicals, fragrances, and exfoliants. Cleansing should be done twice daily with a mild soap or cleanser, followed by a moisturizer.

Diet is also important for maintaining healthy skin. Eating a balanced diet with plenty of fruits, vegetables and proteins helps to nourish the skin from the inside, while limiting sugar and processed foods can help reduce inflammation. Drinking plenty of water helps to keep the skin hydrated. Skin care for aging adults should also include regular skin care routines. Use a gentle exfoliant once a week to remove dead skin cells and help promote cell turnover. Facial masks can help nourish and replenish the skin, while face serums and creams can help reduce fine lines and wrinkles.

Aging skin is more fragile and vulnerable to damage, so it is important to treat it with extra care and attention. Following a consistent skin care routine with appropriate products can help maintain healthy, youthful skin and protect it from damage.

Nail Care

Nail care is an important part of maintaining good health as we age. As we age, our nails become more brittle, dry and prone to splitting, so proper care and attention is essential to keeping them healthy. By taking care of our nails, we can help prevent infections and keep them looking their best.

The most common nail problem in seniors is brittle nails. Brittle nails can be caused by age, dehydration, a lack of vitamins, or a deficiency in calcium or iron. This problem can be managed by using a moisturizing cream or lotion after washing the hands and nails. It is also beneficial to use gloves when washing dishes or cleaning. Additionally, a diet that is rich in calcium, iron, and vitamins can help keep nails strong and healthy. Aging nails can also become discolored, or yellow. This can be caused by smoking, sun exposure, or certain medications. There are several treatments available to help restore the nail's natural color. One option is a nail polish that contains a pigment that matches the natural color of the nails. Alternatively, a nail whitening product can be used to restore the natural color.

Fungal nail infections can also be a problem for seniors. This is caused by a fungus that grows in warm, moist environments and can cause the nails to become thick, yellow, and brittle. To prevent fungal nail infections, it is important to keep the nails clean and dry. If a fungal infection does occur, it can be treated with an antifungal medication.

Splitting nails is another common nail problem in seniors. This can be caused by age, dehydration, or a lack of vitamins and minerals. To prevent splitting nails, it is important to keep the nails moisturized. A moisturizer should be applied after washing the hands and nails, and gloves should be worn when doing housework or gardening. Additionally, a diet that is rich in vitamins and minerals can help keep nails strong and healthy. It is important to remember that nail care is essential to overall health and wellbeing as we age. By taking care of our nails, we can help prevent infections, keep them looking their best, and improve our overall health and wellbeing. With proper care and attention, we can keep our nails healthy and strong even as we age.

CHAPTER THREE

Clothing Basics

Wardrobe for Different Ages

A wardrobe is a very important part of a person's life. It is an expression of who they are, and it can also tell a lot about how they feel. Having the right wardrobe for different ages is important to ensure that people look and feel their best. Depending on the age of a person, their wardrobe should reflect the age-appropriate style and trends.

When it comes to wardrobe for toddlers and young children, comfort is key. They should be dressed in clothes that are easy to move around in and that will keep them warm and protected from the elements. Clothing should be made of breathable fabrics, such as cotton and linen, and should be lightweight and comfortable. Avoid clothing with too many embellishments, as well as any clothing that may be too tight or restrictive. For children, bright colors and fun patterns are always a good choice.

For pre-teens and teenagers, fashion trends become more important. Their wardrobe should reflect the latest trends and styles, but should also be age-appropriate. Clothing should be comfortable, but also stylish. Jeans and t-shirts are always a great choice for teenagers, but they can also experiment with different cuts and colors. Feel free to choose fun patterns and bright colors as well. It is also important to choose clothing that is appropriate for the weather, so always be sure to check the temperature before getting dressed.

For adults, wardrobe choices should be more tailored to their individual style. They should choose clothing that is appropriate for their profession and lifestyle. Businesswear should be professional and should always be tailored to fit well. Avoid clothing that is too tight or too loose. For casual wear, comfort is still important, but adults can also experiment with different trends and styles.

When it comes to wardrobe for seniors, comfort and practicality should be prioritized. Choose clothing that is easy to move in and that is not too tight or restrictive. Clothes should also be appropriate for the weather, and seniors should avoid clothing with too many embellishments or patterns.

No matter what age a person is, wardrobe choices should always reflect their personal style and reflect the current trends. With the right wardrobe, people of all ages can look and feel their best.

Dressing for Different Occasions

Dressing for different occasions can be a daunting task for some people. It is important to know what to wear for different occasions so you look your best and make the right impression.

The first thing to consider when dressing for a different occasion is the type of event. Is it a formal event such as a wedding or a party, or a more casual event such as a picnic or a barbecue? It is important to dress appropriately for the occasion.

For formal events like a wedding or a party, the best options are usually dresses, suits, and evening gowns. For women, a cocktail dress or a dressy evening gown are usually the best options. For men, a suit or a tuxedo is typically the best choice. It is important to keep in mind the color and style of the outfit as well as the accessories. Jewellery and shoes should also be chosen with care to ensure that the overall look is appropriate for the event.

For more casual occasions, such as a picnic or a barbecue, the options are much more varied. For women, the best choices are usually jeans, shorts, and t-shirts. For men, polo shirts and khakis are often appropriate. It is important to keep in mind the weather when choosing an outfit for a casual event. If it is hot outside, a lighter material such as cotton or linen may be more appropriate. When attending a business meeting, the best option is usually a suit. For women, a pencil skirt and blouse or a dressy pantsuit are usually the best choices. For men, a suit and tie is typically the best choice. It is important to make sure the suit is tailored to fit properly and that the overall look is professional. When dressing for a job interview, the best choice is usually a suit. For women, a skirt and blouse or a dressy pantsuit are usually the best options. For men, a suit and tie is typically the best choice. It is important to make sure the suit is tailored to fit properly and that the overall look is professional.

When attending a religious service, the best choice is usually modest attire. For women, a dress or skirt and blouse are usually the best options. For men, a dress shirt and slacks are typically the best choice. It is important to remember that religious services often require more modest attire so it is best to avoid overly revealing clothing.

When dressing for any occasion, it is important to remember to be comfortable and confident. Choose an outfit that makes you feel good and is appropriate for the event. With the right outfit, you can make the best impression and enjoy the event.

Styling Tips for Different Body Types

Aging brings about changes in our bodies that can be difficult to adjust to. Many of us struggle to dress in a way that looks good and is flattering to our new shape. For aging adults, finding the right clothes for your body type can be a challenge, but it doesn't have to be. With a few styling tips, you can look your best no matter your age or body type.

Pear Shaped

For those with a pear shaped body, it is important to choose clothing that will balance out your silhouette. This can be achieved by drawing attention to your upper body and playing down your lower body. To do this, opt for tops with interesting necklines, such as boat necks, scoop necks, and v-necks. Wide leg trousers, A-line skirts, and boot cut jeans can also be used to balance out your shape. For those who prefer dresses, look for ones that are fitted on the top and have an A-line or full skirt.

Apple Shaped

Women with apple shaped bodies should look for clothing that will help to define their waist. Structured blazers, fitted tops, and wrap dresses are great options for this body type. Avoid boxy shapes, as they can make your torso look bigger than it is. Instead, opt for clothing that cinches at the waist to create an hourglass shape. When it comes to bottoms, straight leg trousers and jeans are a good choice, as they balance out the shape of your body.

Rectangle Shaped

For those with a rectangle shape, look for clothing that will create curves. Try opting for items with a cinched waist, such as wrap dresses, belted blazers, and empire-waist tops. Pleated skirts and A-line dresses are also great for creating curves. When it comes to bottoms, try choosing bootcut jeans and flared trousers to add some shape to your outfit.

Hourglass Shaped

If you have an hourglass shape, you're in luck. This body type looks great in almost any type of clothing. To show off your curves, opt for body-hugging pieces such as wrap dresses, pencil skirts, and skinny jeans. If you want to add some volume to your look, try wearing tops with interesting necklines, such as scoop necks and v-necks.

Inverted Triangle Shaped

For those with an inverted triangle shape, look for clothing that will draw attention to the lower half of your body. Try wearing bottoms with interesting details, such as wide leg trousers, boot cut jeans, and A-line skirts. Pair these bottoms with boxier tops and jackets to balance out your silhouette.

No matter what your body type, there are styling tips that can help you look your best. With the right clothes, you can look and feel your best no matter what your age or body type.

CHAPTER FOUR

Accessorizing Basics

Basics of Accessories

When it comes to staying active and healthy, accessories are an important part of the equation for aging adults. Accessories can help an aging senior stay safe, independent, and comfortable. They can also make everyday tasks easier, help seniors stay active, and improve their overall quality of life.

Safety accessories are an important consideration for aging adults. This includes items like grab bars, shower chairs, and raised toilet seats, which can help prevent falls in the bathroom. Mobility aids, such as canes, walkers, and wheelchairs, can help seniors stay mobile and independent. They can also reduce fatigue and help seniors maintain their balance. Safety accessories can also include assistive devices like hearing aids and eyeglasses, which can help seniors stay connected with their environment.

Comfort accessories can also be important for aging adults. Items like orthopedic shoes, cushioned insoles, and foot supports can help reduce pain and provide support for the feet. Pillows, mattress toppers, and specialty beds can also help improve comfort and reduce the risk of pressure sores. Items like compression garments can help reduce swelling in the legs and improve circulation.

Accessories can also be used to help aging adults stay active and engaged. Exercise accessories such as hand weights, balance balls, and resistance bands can help seniors stay fit and toned. Cognitive accessories, such as puzzles and games, can help keep seniors mentally sharp and engaged. In addition to the physical and mental benefits they provide, accessories can also help seniors stay socially active. Video calling devices, such as Skype or FaceTime, can help seniors stay connected with family and friends. Music players, such as iPods and MP3 players, can help seniors enjoy their favorite tunes.

When it comes to staying safe, comfortable, and active, accessories are an important part of the equation for aging adults. From safety accessories, to comfort accessories, to cognitive and exercise aids, there are a variety of items that can help seniors stay healthy and independent. With the right accessories, seniors can stay active, engaged, and connected, and enjoy a better quality of life.

Accessories for Different Ages

Accessories for different ages are the perfect way to express yourself and make a statement. Whether it is a child, a teenager, or an adult, there are a variety of accessories that can be used to show off your unique style and personality. Accessories can range from jewelry, hats, bags, and belts to shoes, scarves, and sunglasses. It is important to choose the right accessories to fit your age because the wrong choice can make you look out of place.

For children, accessories are an opportunity to show off their unique style. They can choose from a variety of colorful and fun items such as hats, bags, and jewelry. Parents should ensure that their children's accessories are age appropriate and are not too flashy or ostentatious. Accessories should also be chosen to suit their individual personalities. For example, a young girl may prefer a bright and bold necklace or earrings, while a boy may prefer a subtler and understated hat.

Teenagers often like to experiment with different styles and accessories. They may choose to wear items that are more daring or edgy than those of younger children. Popular accessories for teenagers include statement jewelry, hats, scarves, and sunglasses. These items can be used to make a bold statement and express their individual style. Adults can also express their unique style through accessories. They may choose items such as watches, wallets, and ties to complete their look. Accessories for adults should be chosen to match their clothing and reflect their personality. For example, a sophisticated adult may choose to wear a classic watch or a stylish tie.

No matter what age you are, accessories are a great way to express yourself and make a statement. When selecting accessories, it is important to choose items that are age appropriate and match your style. Whether you are a child, a teenager, or an adult, there are a variety of accessories that can be used to show off your unique personality. So go ahead and accessorize!

Accessorizing for Different Occasions

Accessorizing is an essential part of any outfit, and accessorizing for different occasions can be quite difficult. The right accessories can make or break an outfit, so it's important to consider the occasion when picking out pieces. With so many different occasions and styles to consider, it can be helpful to break it down into categories.

Casual Outings

For casual outings, the most important thing is to keep it simple. Jeans and a T-shirt are always a classic combination, and they can easily be dressed up or down with the right accessories. A great way to add a bit of pizzazz is to choose statement jewelry pieces. A bold necklace or earrings can really draw attention to an outfit. A great bag is also a must-have for any casual ensemble. Choose a bag in a bright color or an eye-catching pattern to really make a statement.

Formal Events

When dressing for a formal event, you may need to pull out all the stops. A formal dress is a great way to make a statement, and the accessories you choose can really put the look over the top. For example, a pair of sparkly earrings or a necklace with a bit of bling can make any dress look more glamorous. Similarly, a clutch or evening bag in a bright color or striking pattern can add an extra touch of elegance. When it comes to shoes, choose a daring pair of heels to really make the look stand out.

Work Attire

When it comes to work attire, the goal is to look polished and professional. While it may be tempting to go all out with accessories, it's important to keep it toned down. Classic jewelry pieces such as stud earrings, a simple necklace, and a watch are great options. For a bag, choose a practical yet stylish one that will fit everything you need for the day. As for shoes, opt for a pair of classic pumps or loafers to complete the look.

Beachwear

Beachwear is all about having fun and making a statement. A great way to accessorize a beach outfit is with a pair of statement sunglasses. Choose a bright color or a unique shape to really make an impact. Similarly, a colorful hat or a fun beach bag can really liven up the look. When it comes to jewelry, opt for pieces with a beachy vibe, such as shells or starfish. Finally, don't forget your sandals! Choose a pair of stylish sandals or flip flops to complete the look.

No matter what the occasion, accessorizing is a great way to take an outfit to the next level. By considering the event and the type of outfit you're wearing, you can easily choose the right accessories to make your look complete.

CHAPTER FIVE

Makeup Basics

Basics of Makeup

Makeup is a form of art that can enhance and improve the beauty of an individual. It can be used to create a variety of looks, from subtle and natural to dramatic and glamorous. Makeup is an important part of a woman's beauty routine, and can be a great way to express your individual style.

The first step to applying makeup is to prepare your skin. This involves cleansing your face with a gentle cleanser, exfoliating to remove dead skin cells, and moisturizing to keep your skin hydrated. This will help to ensure that your makeup will last all day and keep your skin looking healthy.

Once your skin is ready, it's time to begin applying makeup. The most basic makeup routine involves applying foundation, concealer, and powder.

Foundation is a creamy product that is used to even out skin tone and provide a base for the rest of your makeup. Concealer is a thicker product that is used to cover blemishes and dark circles. Powder is used to set the makeup and prevent it from smudging or creasing.

Next, you can add color to your face with blush, bronzer, and highlighter. Blush is a powder or cream product used to add a natural flush to the cheeks. Bronzer is a powder or cream used to add a warm glow to the skin. Highlighter is a shimmery powder used to highlight the highest points of the face.

Once you have your foundation, blush, bronzer, and highlighter applied, you can move on to eye makeup. Eye makeup consists of eyeshadow, eyeliner, and mascara. Eyeshadow is a powder used to create depth and color on the eyelid. Eyeliner is a pencil or liquid product used to line the eyes and create a variety of looks. Mascara is a liquid product used to add length and volume to the lashes.

Finally, you can add lipstick, lip liner, and lip gloss. Lipstick is a creamy product used to add color and definition to the lips. Lip liner is a pencil product used to outline and define the shape of the lips. Lip gloss is a sheer product used to add shine and moisture to the lips.

Makeup is an art form that can help to enhance and improve an individual's appearance. It is important to take the time to find the right products and colors that work best for you. With practice and patience, you can create a variety of looks to fit any occasion.

Makeup for Different Ages

Makeup is an essential part of any woman's beauty routine, regardless of age. While many women in their teens and twenties rely on makeup to give them a youthful glow, older women may prefer to use makeup to enhance their features and minimize the signs of aging. It is important to understand the makeup tips and tricks that are best suited to different ages so that you can look your best. For younger women, the emphasis should be on accentuating the features they already have and creating a natural, youthful look. One of the best ways to achieve this is by using products with light, natural colors such as peach, pink, and beige. It is also important to use makeup to create the illusion of a more defined jawline, to make the eyes appear larger, and to give the lips a fuller, more defined look.

For women in their thirties and forties, the focus should be on creating a more polished and mature look. This can be achieved by using foundation and concealer to even out the skin tone and create a more even complexion. Eye shadows in shades of brown and gray can be used to create a smoky eye look, while blushes in shades of pink and peach can be used to add a flush of color to the cheeks. For women in their fifties and sixties, makeup should be used to minimize the signs of aging. This can be done by using foundation and concealer to cover up any fine lines or wrinkles. To add a bit of a youthful glow to the skin, opt for a luminous foundation or a tinted moisturizer. For the eyes, use light, neutral colors to make them appear more open and bright. Blush should be used sparingly, as it can easily make the face look overly made up.

No matter what age you are, it is important to take care of your skin in order to ensure that your makeup looks its best. Make sure to use a gentle cleanser, moisturizer, and sunscreen to keep your skin looking healthy and vibrant. Additionally, make sure to use makeup remover to remove all traces of makeup before going to bed.

In conclusion, makeup is an essential part of any woman's beauty routine, regardless of age. With the right tips and tricks, you can create a look that is perfect for your age and that makes you look and feel your best. From light and natural colors for younger women to products that minimize the signs of aging for older women, there are plenty of options available to help you look your best.

Makeup for Different Occasions

Makeup is a great way to enhance your look for different occasions. Whether you are going to a formal event or a casual day out, makeup can help you create the perfect look.

For formal events, makeup should be applied to create a polished and sophisticated look. Start by applying a foundation that matches your skin tone, then use a concealer to cover any blemishes or dark circles. Finish off the base with a light dusting of powder and a blush to give your cheeks a natural flush. Then, you can use a combination of eyeshadows, eyeliners, and mascaras to create a dramatic eye look. Finally, finish off your look with a bold lipstick or lip gloss to complete the look.

For casual occasions, makeup should be kept more natural. Start by applying a light foundation and concealer, then add a finishing powder. Use a bronzer to warm up your complexion and a light blush to add a touch of color. Don't overdo it with eyeshadows and eyeliners, instead opt for a subtle cat eye look with a few coats of mascara. Finish off the look with a natural lip color or a light tinted lip balm.

When attending a wedding, opt for a romantic and ethereal makeup look. Start by applying a foundation that matches your skin tone, then use a concealer to cover any blemishes or dark circles. Finish off the base with a light dusting of powder and a blush to give your cheeks a natural flush. Then, use a combination of light and shimmery eyeshadows and eyeliners to create a romantic look. Finally, finish off your look with a bold lip color to complete the look.

No matter the event, makeup can help you create the perfect look. Whether you are attending a formal event or a casual day out, there are makeup looks to suit every occasion. Start with a foundation that matches your skin tone, then use a concealer to cover any blemishes or dark circles.

Finish off the base with a light dusting of powder and a blush to give your cheeks a natural flush. Then, use a combination of eyeshadows, eyeliners, and mascaras to create the perfect eye look. Finally, finish off the look with a bold lip color or a light tinted lip balm to complete the look.

CHAPTER SIX

Grooming and Styling Tips

Tips for Looking Younger

Looking younger can be a daunting task, but it doesn't have to be. With the right tips and tricks, you can easily look younger and more refreshed. From simple lifestyle changes to more advanced treatments, these tips will help you look younger and more vibrant.

1. Wear Sunscreen: Sun damage can age your skin quickly, so it's important to protect yourself from the sun's damaging rays. Make sure to wear sunscreen every day, even when it's cloudy. Choose a broad-spectrum sunscreen with an SPF of at least 15, and reapply it throughout the day.

2. Moisturize: Keeping your skin hydrated is key to looking younger and more vibrant. Moisturize your skin twice a day and make sure to choose a moisturizer that is right for your skin type.

3. Use Retinoids: Retinoids are a type of vitamin A that can help reduce the appearance of wrinkles and fine lines. Retinoids are available over the counter or by prescription, so talk to your doctor or dermatologist about which one is right for you.

4. Eat Well: Eating a healthy, balanced diet can help you look younger and more vibrant. Make sure to eat plenty of fruits and vegetables, whole grains, and lean proteins. Avoid processed foods and sugary snacks, as they can age your skin.

5. Exercise: Exercise is important for your overall health, but it can also help you look younger. Exercise can help improve circulation and reduce wrinkles. Aim for 30 minutes of exercise per day, such as walking, jogging, or swimming.

6. Get Enough Sleep: Lack of sleep can age your skin, so make sure to get at least seven to nine hours of sleep each night.

7. Avoid Stress: Stress can cause wrinkles and other signs of aging, so try to reduce stress in your life. Practice relaxation techniques such as yoga, meditation, or deep breathing.

8. Use Antioxidants: Antioxidants can help reduce signs of aging by fighting off free radicals. Look for products that contain antioxidants such as vitamin C, green tea, or resveratrol.

9. Use Facial Oils: Facial oils can help keep your skin hydrated and youthful. Choose an oil that is right for your skin type, such as argan or jojoba oil.

10. Use Facial Masks: Facial masks can help reduce wrinkles and other signs of aging. Look for masks that contain natural ingredients such as aloe vera, honey, or avocado.

11. See a Dermatologist: If you're looking for a more advanced treatment, make sure to see a dermatologist. A dermatologist can help you decide which treatments are right for you, such as chemical peels, microdermabrasion, or laser treatments.

These are just a few tips for looking younger. With the right lifestyle changes and treatments, you can look younger and more vibrant. Talk to your doctor or dermatologist about which treatments are right for you.

Tips for Looking Professional

The way you look can greatly influence the way people perceive you and can be a key factor in how successful you are in your professional life. Looking professional is essential in any profession, from entry-level positions to executive roles. There are several tips for looking professional that can help you make a great first impression and be taken seriously in any situation.

One of the most important tips for looking professional is to dress for the occasion. It is important to be aware of the dress code of your company or the event you are attending. Make sure you are wearing clothing that is appropriate for the occasion and is appropriate for the job.

Avoid wearing clothing that is too casual or too formal. Make sure to accessorize appropriately and avoid wearing too much jewelry or makeup.

Another important tip for looking professional is to maintain good hygiene. Make sure to shower, comb your hair, and brush your teeth regularly. It is also important to wear deodorant and use a light cologne or perfume. If you wear makeup, make sure it looks natural and is not too heavy.

It is also important to maintain good posture when interacting with people. Make sure to stand straight, make eye contact, and smile when appropriate. Pay attention to your body language and make sure it is positive. Avoid crossing your arms or slouching as this can give off a negative impression.

Another tip for looking professional is to be well groomed. Make sure your hair is neat and combed and your nails are trimmed. It is also important to be conscious of any facial hair or stubble and make sure it looks neat.

Finally, it is important to carry yourself in a confident manner. Make sure to speak clearly and avoid using slang or crude language. Make sure to practice good manners and be polite. Make sure to be aware of the conversation and contribute when appropriate.

By following these tips for looking professional, you can make a great first impression and be taken seriously in any professional situation. Being aware of appropriate dress codes and practicing good hygiene, posture, grooming, and manners are essential for looking professional. With a little effort and practice, you can make sure you are looking professional in any situation.

Tips for Looking Stylish

When it comes to looking stylish, there are no hard and fast rules. Everyone has their own style and it is important to find the one that makes you feel confident and comfortable. With that being said, there are a few tips that can help you look stylish no matter what your personal style is.

First, it is important to invest in quality pieces. Quality pieces are an investment that will last and look better over time. Investing in quality pieces will not only make you look stylish, but it will also help you save money in the long run.

Second, it is important to find a way to make your wardrobe look cohesive. This can be done by creating a color palette that you can use when you are shopping. This way, you can ensure all of the pieces you buy will look great together. You can also find ways to mix and match different pieces to create different looks.

Third, it is important to have pieces that can be dressed up or down. Having a few key pieces that you can dress up or down will make it easier for you to create multiple looks with your wardrobe.

Fourth, it is important to accessorize. Accessories can make any outfit look more stylish. A few key pieces like a statement necklace, a scarf, or a hat can take an ordinary outfit and make it look more put together.

Fifth, it is important to take care of your clothes. Taking care of your clothes will help them last longer and look better for longer. Investing in quality pieces is important, but it is also important to make sure you are taking care of those pieces.

Finally, it is important to wear clothes that fit properly. Wearing clothes that fit properly will not only make you look more stylish but it will also help you feel more confident.

These are just a few tips that can help you look stylish no matter what your personal style is. Remember that looking stylish is not about following trends, it is about creating a look that is unique to you. Find pieces that make you feel confident and comfortable and you will be sure to look stylish.

CHAPTER SEVEN

Conclusion

Summary

Aging adults are a rapidly growing demographic in the United States. The population of Americans aged 65 and older is projected to double by the year 2030, growing from 48 million in 2018 to an estimated 98 million. This population growth has major implications for society, and it is important to understand the facts about aging adults in order to best support them.

The most notable fact about aging adults is that they are living longer. The life expectancy for a person in the United States is now 78.6 years, up from 75.2 years in 1990. In addition, the number of people aged 85 and older is expected to nearly triple by 2050, increasing from 6 million to 16 million. Aging adults also face a higher risk of chronic conditions. By age 65, seven out of ten Americans have at least one chronic condition, such as diabetes, heart disease, or arthritis. In addition, a large portion of aging adults will experience some form of cognitive decline, such as dementia or Alzheimer's disease. Aging adults are also more likely to experience social isolation. This is especially true for those living alone, who make up nearly one-third of the over 65 populations. Social isolation can have serious consequences, as loneliness and depression can lead to an increased risk of cognitive decline and other health issues.

Finally, aging adults are also more likely to experience financial hardship. Those aged 65 and older are more likely to live on a fixed income, making it difficult for them to afford basic necessities. In addition, many aging adults are unable to access the resources they need to remain healthy and active, such as transportation and medical care. These facts about aging adults demonstrate the need for society to better support this population. This includes providing access to affordable housing, transportation, and health care, as well as programs that help aging adults stay connected with their communities. It also means being aware of the signs of social isolation and providing interventions to help aging adults stay healthy and connected.

By understanding the facts about aging adults, we can create a society that is better equipped to support this growing population. With the right resources and support, aging adults can look forward to a healthy and fulfilling life.

Final Thoughts

Aging is a natural process that affects all adults, and the effects of aging can be both positive and negative. While aging brings with it a certain amount of frailty, it can also bring wisdom, insight, and a greater appreciation for life. It is important to remember that aging is a process, and there is no one-size-fits-all approach to dealing with aging adults. Each individual's experience of aging will be unique and will vary depending on their physical, emotional, and social circumstances.

One of the most important facts about aging adults is that they will experience a decrease in physical strength and mobility. This is a normal part of aging and can be managed with appropriate exercise and physical activity. In addition, aging adults are often more prone to chronic health conditions such as arthritis, heart disease, and diabetes. Early detection and treatment of these conditions can help to reduce the impact of aging on an individual's life.

Another important fact about aging adults is that they may experience changes in cognitive functioning, such as a reduction in memory and concentration. This is a normal part of aging and can be managed with appropriate lifestyle choices and mental health support. For example, engaging in mentally stimulating activities, such as puzzles and games, can help to maintain cognitive functioning. It is also important for aging adults to receive adequate social support, as this can help to reduce feelings of loneliness and isolation.

Finally, it is important to remember that aging adults should be encouraged to maintain a positive outlook on life. This can be achieved through meaningful activities, such as volunteering or engaging in creative hobbies. Maintaining social contact with family and friends is also important, as it can help to provide a sense of connection and purpose.

In conclusion, aging is an inevitable part of life and can be a difficult process for many adults. However, with the right support and lifestyle choices, aging adults can continue to live fulfilling and meaningful lives. It is important to remember that each person's experience of aging will be unique and to provide the necessary support and care to help aging adults live as independently as possible.